Keto Diet for Weight Loss

A cookbook of Tasty recipes to lose weight easily while continuing to eat the foods you love!

Dana Roberts

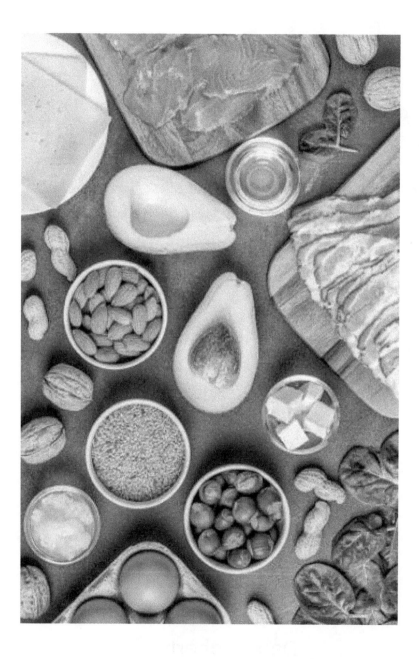

Table of contents

Quick Recipes   9

    Quinoa Bowls   10

    Cornmeal Porridge   12

    Breakfast Rice Pudding   14

    Breakfast Tortillas   16

    Special Pancake   18

    Millet and Oats Porridge   20

Lunch Recipes   23

    Eggs Benedict Deviled Eggs   24

    Spinach Meatballs   26

    Bacon Wrapped Asparagus   28

    Buttered Cod   30

    Chicken and Rice Congee   32

    Steamed Cod with Ginger   34

    Flounder with Dill and Capers   36

    Chili-Garlic Salmon   38

    Chili-Lime Shrimps   40

    Tuna Patties   42

    Grilled Mahi Mahi with Lemon Butter Sauce   44

    Shrimp Scampi   46

Dinner Recipes   49

    Quick Pumpkin Soup   50

    Fresh Avocado Soup   52

    Creamy Garlic Chicken   54

    Garlicky Pork Shoulder   56

Rosemary Pork Roast	58
Persian Chicken	60
Pesto Pork Chops	62
Roasted Red Pepper and Eggplant Soup	64
Cilantro-Lime Flounder	66
Dessert Recipes	69
Snickerdoodle Muffins	70
Egg Custard	72
Mocha Ice Cream	74
Condiment Recipes	77
Thai Peanut Sauce	78
General Tso Sauce	80
Smoothies Recipes	83
Tropical Green Paleo Smoothie	84
Vegan Banana Avocado Green Smoothie Bowl with Blueberries	86
Kale Strawberry Green Smoothie Bowl	88
Salad Recipes	91
Potluck Lamb Salad	92
Spring Supper Salad	94
Chicken-of-Sea Salad	96
Sweet Potato Salad	98
Appetizers and Snacks	101
Spiced Jalapeno Bites with Tomato	102
Coconut Crab Cakes	104
Tuna Cakes	106
Tempura Zucchini with Cream Cheese Dip	108

Bacon and Feta Skewers   110

Avocado and Prosciutto Deviled Eggs   112

Chicken Club Lettuce Wraps   114

About the author   118

Dana Roberts

Quick Recipes

Quinoa Bowls

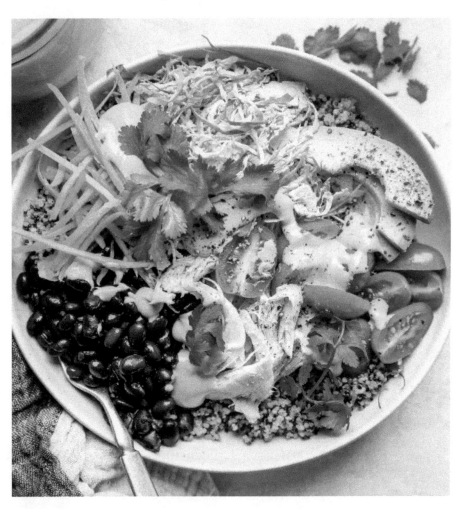

Preparation time: 10 Minutes

Cooking time: 1 Minute

Servings: 4

Ingredients:

- 1 and ½ Cups quinoa
- 2 Tablespoons honey
- 2 and ¼ Cups of water
- ¼ Teaspoon pumpkin pie spice
- 2 Cups strawberries, chopped

Directions:

1. In your instant pot, mix quinoa with honey, water, spice, and strawberries, stir, cover, and cook on high for 1 minute.
2. Leave quinoa aside for 10 minutes, stir a bit, divide everything into bowls and serve.
3. Enjoy!

Nutrition:

- Calories: 162
- Fat: 3
- Fiber: 3
- Carbs: 6
- Protein: 3

Cornmeal Porridge

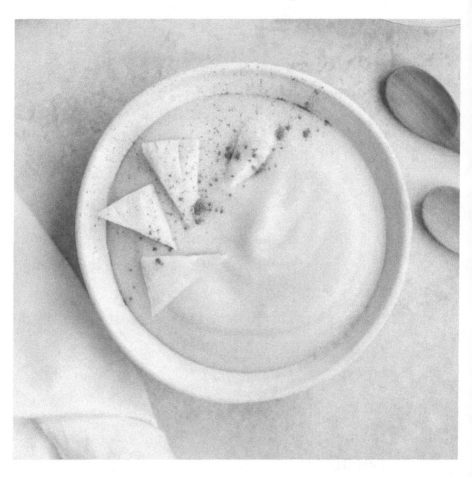

Preparation time: 10 Minutes

Cooking time: 20 Minutes

Servings: 4

Ingredients:

- 1 Cup cornmeal
- 1 Cup milk
- 4 Cups of water
- ½ Teaspoon nutmeg, ground
- ½ Cup sweetened condensed milk

Directions:

1. In a bowl, mix 1 cup water with cornmeal and stir well.
2. In your instant pot, mix the rest of the water with milk and cornmeal mix and stir.
3. Also, add nutmeg, stir, cover, and cook on high for 6 minutes.
4. Add condensed milk, stir, divide into bowls, and serve.
5. Enjoy!

Nutrition:

- Calories: 241 Fat: 4
- Fiber: 6 Carbs: 12
- Protein: 6

Breakfast Rice Pudding

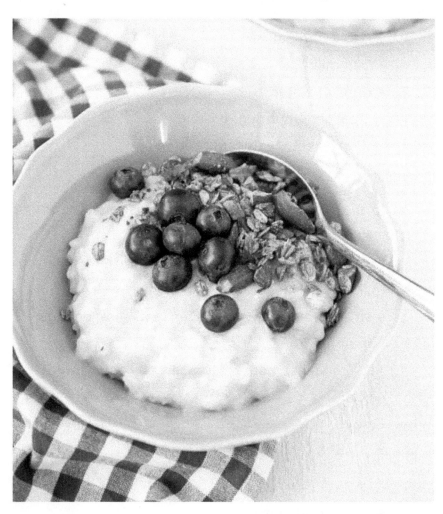

Preparation time: 10 Minutes

Cooking time: 20 Minutes

Servings: 6

Ingredients:

- 2 Cups nut milk
- 1 and ¼ Cups water
- 1 Cup basmati rice
- 1 Cup coconut cream
- ¼ Cup maple syrup

Directions:

1. In your instant pot, mix nut milk with water, rice, cream, and maple syrup, stir well, cover, and cook on high for 20 minutes.
2. Stir pudding again, divide into bowls and serve.
3. Enjoy!

Nutrition:

- Calories: 251
- Fat: 5
- Fiber: 3
- Carbs: 6
- Protein: 5

Breakfast Tortillas

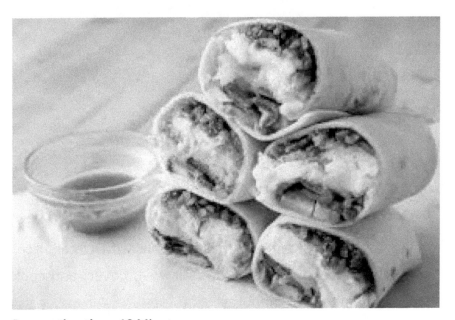

Preparation time: 10 Minutes

Cooking time: 13 Minutes

Servings: 6

Ingredients:

- 2 Pounds red potatoes, cubed
- 4 Eggs, whisked
- 6 Ounces ham, cubed
- ¼ Cup yellow onion, chopped

For the instant pot:

- 1 Cup water

For Serving:

- 6 Tortillas

Directions:

1. In a bowl, mix eggs with ham, onion, and potatoes and whisk well.
2. Add this to a baking dish and spread.
3. Add water to your instant pot, add trivet, add baking dish inside, cover and cook on high for 13 minutes.
4. Arrange tortillas on a working surface, divide eggs, mix on each, wrap and serve for breakfast.
5. Enjoy!

Nutrition:

- Calories: 212
- Fat: 3
- Fiber: 7
- Carbs: 9
- Protein: 12

Special Pancake

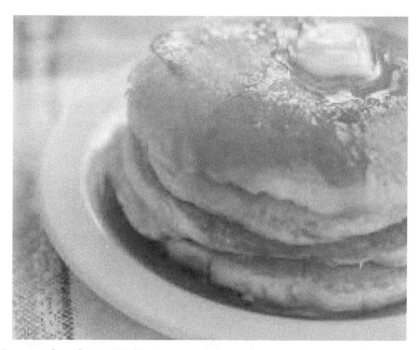

Preparation time: 10 Minutes

Cooking time: 45 Minutes

Servings: 4

Ingredients:

- 2 Cups white flour
- 2 Eggs
- 1 and ½ Cups milk
- 2 Tablespoons sugar
- 2 and ½ Teaspoons baking powder

Directions:

1. In a bowl, mix flour with eggs, milk, sugar, and baking powder and whisk really well.
2. Add this to your instant pot, spread, cover, and cook on Manual for 45 minutes.
3. Leave your pancake to cool down, slice, divide between plates, and serve.
4. Enjoy!

Nutrition:

- Calories: 251
- Fat: 5
- Fiber: 2
- Carbs: 6
- Protein: 3

Millet and Oats Porridge

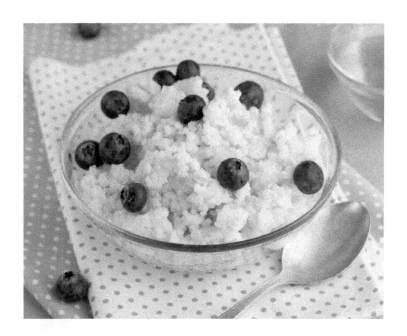

Preparation time: 10 Minutes

Cooking time: 13 Minutes

Servings: 8

Ingredients:

- 1 Cup millet
- ½ Cup rolled oats
- 3 Cups water
- ½ Teaspoon ginger powder
- 2 Apples, cored and chopped

Directions:

1. Set your instant pot on sauté mode, add millet, stir and toast for 3 minutes.
2. Add oats, water, ginger, and apples, stir, cover, and cook on high for 10 minutes.
3. Stir porridge again and divide it into bowls to serve.
4. Enjoy!

Nutrition:

- Calories: 200
- Fat: 2
- Fiber: 3
- Carbs: 4
- Protein: 5

Lunch Recipes

Eggs Benedict Deviled Eggs

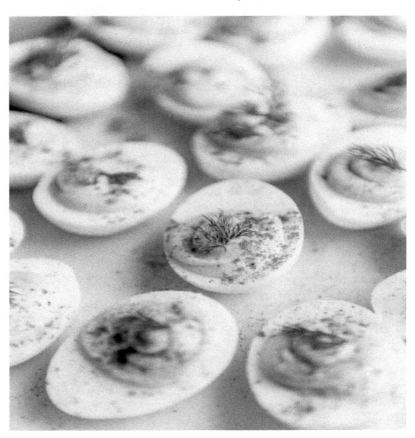

Preparation time: 15 Minutes

Cooking time: 25 Minutes

Servings: 16

Ingredients:

- 8 Hardboiled eggs, sliced in half
- 1 Tablespoon lemon juice
- ½ Teaspoon mustard powder

- 1 Pack Hollandaise sauce mix, prepared according to the directions in the packaging
- 1 lb. Asparagus, trimmed and steamed
- 4oz. Bacon, cooked and chopped

Directions:

1. Scoop out the egg yolks.
2. Mix the egg yolks with lemon juice, mustard powder, and 1/3 cup of the Hollandaise sauce.
3. Spoon the egg yolk mixture into each of the egg whites.
4. Arrange the asparagus spears on a serving plate. Top with the deviled eggs.
5. Sprinkle remaining sauce and bacon on top.

Nutrition:

- Calories: 80 Total Fat: 5.3g
- Saturated Fat: 1.7g Cholesterol: 90mg
- Sodium: 223mg Total Carbohydrate: 2.1g
- Dietary Fiber: 0.6g Total Sugars: 0.7g
- Protein: 6.2g Potassium: 133mg

Spinach Meatballs

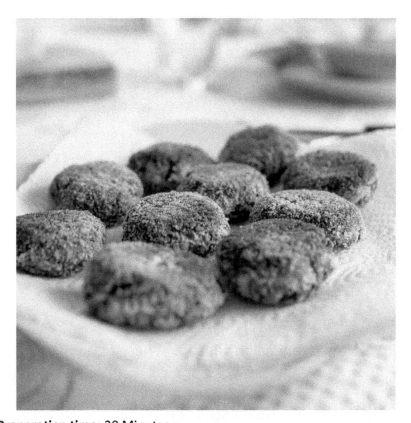

Preparation time: 20 Minutes

Cooking time: 30 Minutes

Servings: 4

Ingredients:

- 1 Cup spinach, chopped
- 1 ½ lb. Ground turkey breast
- 1 Onion, chopped
- 3 Cloves garlic, minced

- 1 Egg, beaten
- ¼ Cup milk
- ¾ Cup breadcrumbs
- ½ Cup Parmesan cheese, grated
- Salt and pepper to taste
- 2 Tablespoons butter
- 2 Tablespoons Keto flour
- 10oz. Italian cheese, shredded
- ½ Teaspoon nutmeg, freshly grated
- ¼ Cup parsley, chopped

Directions:

1. Preheat your oven to 400 degrees F.
2. Mix all the ingredients in a large bowl.
3. Form meatballs from the mixture.
4. Bake in the oven for 20 minutes.

Nutrition:

- Calories: 374 Total Fat: 18.5g
- Saturated Fat: 10g Cholesterol: 118mg
- Sodium: 396mg
- Total Carbohydrate: 11.3g
- Dietary Fiber: 1g Total Sugars: 1.7g
- Protein: 34.2g Potassium: 336mg

Bacon Wrapped Asparagus

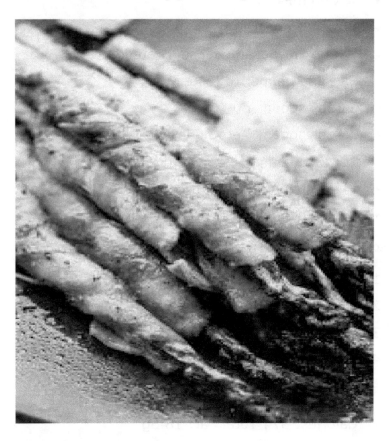

Preparation time: 10 Minutes

Cooking time: 20 Minutes

Servings: 6

Ingredients:

- 1 ½ lb. Asparagus spears, sliced in half
- 6 Slices bacon

- 2 Tablespoons olive oil
- Salt and pepper to taste

Directions:

1. Preheat your oven to 400 degrees F.
2. Wrap a handful of asparagus with bacon.
3. Secure with a toothpick. Drizzle with the olive oil. Season with salt and pepper.
4. Bake in the oven for 20 minutes or until bacon is crispy.

Nutrition:

- Calories: 166 Total Fat: 12.8g
- Saturated Fat: 3.3g Cholesterol: 21mg
- Sodium: 441mg Total Carbohydrate: 4.7g
- Dietary Fiber: 2.4g Total Sugars: 2.1g
- Protein: 9.5g Potassium: 337mg

Buttered Cod

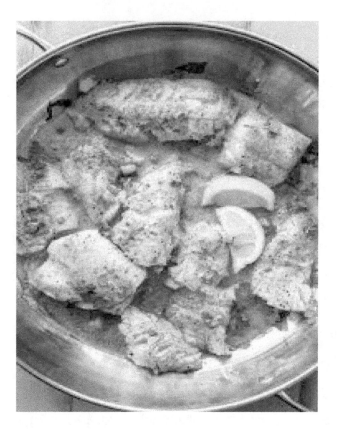

Preparation time: 5 Minutes

Cooking time: 5 Minutes

Servings: 4

Ingredients:

- 1 ½ lb. Cod fillets, sliced
- 6 Tablespoons butter, sliced
- ¼ Teaspoon garlic powder

- ¾ Teaspoon ground paprika
- Salt and pepper to taste
- Lemon slices - Chopped parsley

Directions:

1. Mix the garlic powder, paprika, salt, and pepper in a bowl.
2. Season codpieces with seasoning mixture.
3. Add two tablespoons of butter in a pan over medium heat. Let half of the butter melt. Add the cod and cook for 2 minutes per side. Top with the remaining slices of butter.
4. Cook for 3 to 4 minutes.
5. Garnish with parsley and lemon slices before serving.

Nutrition:

- Calories: 295 Total Fat: 19g
- Saturated Fat: 11g Cholesterol: 128mg
- Sodium: 236mg Total Carbohydrate: 1.5g
- Dietary Fiber: 0.7g Total Sugars: 0.3g
- Protein: 30.7g Potassium: 102mg

Chicken and Rice Congee

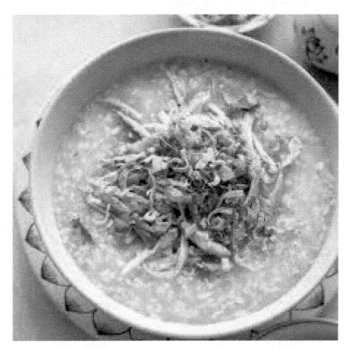

Preparation time: 10 Minutes

Cooking time: 35 Minutes

Servings: 1

Ingredients:

- 90 Grams of rice, brown
- 2 Cups cold water
- 2 Chicken drumsticks
- ½ Tablespoon ginger, sliced into strips
- Salt, to taste

Directions:

1. First, rinse the rice under tap water by gently scrubbing the rice.
2. Drain any milky water. The next step is to add ginger, rice, chicken drumsticks, and water to the instant pot.
3. Do not add salt at this stage.
4. Now close the lid of the pot and cook on high pressure for 30 minutes.
5. Then, naturally, release the steam.
6. Open the lid carefully; check if the congee looks watery. Heat up the instant pot by pressing the sauté button.
7. Cook until the desired thickness is obtained. Season it with salt and then use a fork to separate the meat from the bone.
8. Remove the congee from the pot. Serve and enjoy.

Nutrition:

- Calories: 493 Total Fat: 6g
- Sodium: 248mg
- Total Carbohydrate: 73.9g
- Protein: 32g

Steamed Cod with Ginger

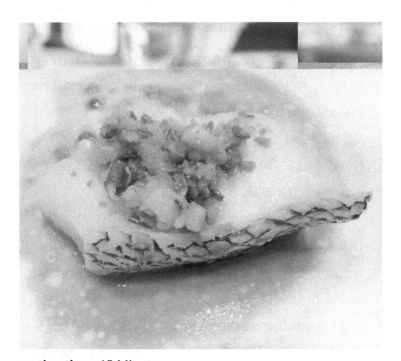

Preparation time: 15 Minutes

Cooking time: 15 Minutes

Servings: 4

Ingredients:

- 4 Cod fillets, skin removed
- 3 Tbsp. lemon juice, freshly squeezed
- 2 Tbsp. coconut aminos
- 2 Tbsp. grated ginger
- 6 Scallions, chopped

Directions:

1. Place a trivet in a large saucepan and pour a cup or two of water into the pan. Bring to a boil.
2. In a small bowl, whisk well lemon juice, coconut aminos, coconut oil, and grated ginger.
3. Place scallions in a heatproof dish that fits inside a saucepan. Season scallion's mon with pepper and salt. Drizzle with ginger mixture. Sprinkle scallions on top.
4. Seal dish with foil. Place the dish on the trivet inside the saucepan—cover and steam for 15 minutes.
5. Serve and enjoy.

Nutrition:

- Calories: 514 Fat: 40g
- Carbohydrates: 10g Protein: 28.3g

Flounder with Dill and Capers

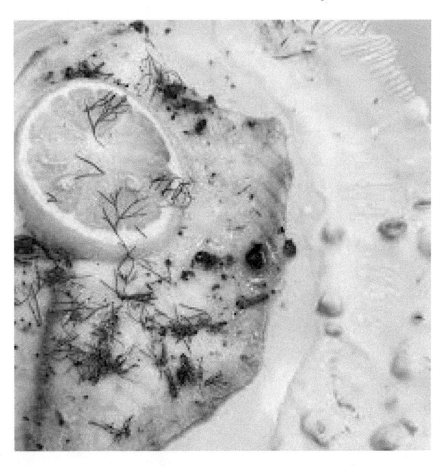

Preparation time: 10 Minutes

Cooking time: 15 Minutes

Servings: 4

Ingredients:

- 4 Flounder fillets
- 1 Tbsp. chopped fresh dill
- 2 Tbsp. capers, chopped
- 4 Lemon wedges

Directions:

1. Place a trivet in a large saucepan and pour a cup or two of water into the pan. Bring to a boil.
2. Place flounder in a heatproof dish that fits inside a saucepan. Season snapper with pepper and salt. Drizzle with olive oil on all sides. Sprinkle dill and capers on top of the filet. Seal dish with foil. Place the dish on the trivet inside the saucepan—cover and steam for 15 minutes.
3. Serve and enjoy with lemon wedges.

Nutrition:

- Calories: 447 Fat: 35.9g
- Carbohydrates: 8.6g Protein: 20.3g

Chili-Garlic Salmon

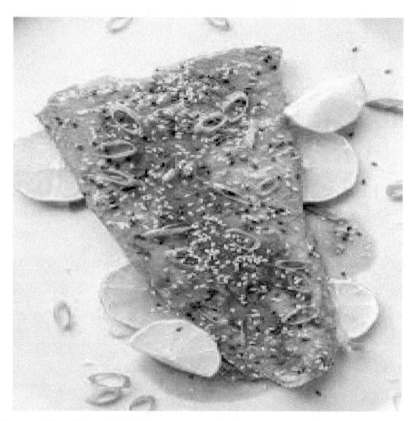

Preparation time: 10 Minutes

Cooking time: 15 Minutes

Servings: 4

Ingredients:

- 5 Tbsp. sweet chili sauce
- ¼ Cup coconut aminos

- 4 Salmon fillets
- 3 Tbsp. green onions, chopped
- 3 Cloves garlic, peeled and minced

Directions:

1. Place a trivet in a large saucepan and pour a cup or two of water into the pan. Bring to a boil.
2. In a small bowl, whisk well sweet chili sauce, garlic, and coconut aminos.
3. Place salmon in a heatproof dish that fits inside a saucepan. Season salmon with pepper. Drizzle with sweet chili sauce mixture. Sprinkle green onions on top of the filet.
4. Seal dish with foil. Place the dish on the trivet inside the saucepan. Cover and steam for 15 minutes.
5. Serve and enjoy.

Nutrition:

- Calories: 409 Fat: 14.4g
- Carbohydrates: 0.9g Protein: 65.4g

Chili-Lime Shrimps

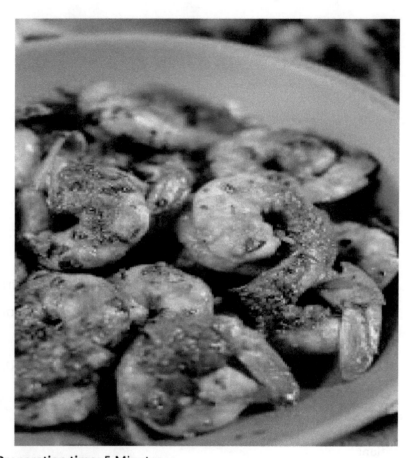

Preparation time: 5 Minutes

Cooking time: 10 Minutes

Servings: 4

Ingredients:

- 1 ½ lb. Raw shrimp, peeled and deveined
- 1 Tbsp. chili flakes
- 5 Tbsp sweet chili sauce

- 2 Tbsp. lime juice, freshly squeezed
- 1 Tsp. cayenne pepper

Directions:

1. In a small bowl, whisk well chili flakes, sweet chili sauce, cayenne pepper, and water.
2. On medium-high fire, heat a non-stick saucepan for 2 minutes. Add oil to a pan and swirl to coat the bottom and sides—heat the oil for a minute.
3. Stir fry shrimp, around 5 minutes. Season lightly with salt and pepper.
4. Stir in sweet chili mixture and toss well shrimp to coat.
5. Turn off fire, drizzle lime juice and toss well to coat.
6. Serve and enjoy.

Nutrition:

- Calories: 306 Fat: 19.8g
- Carbohydrates: 1.7g Protein: 34.9.g

Tuna Patties

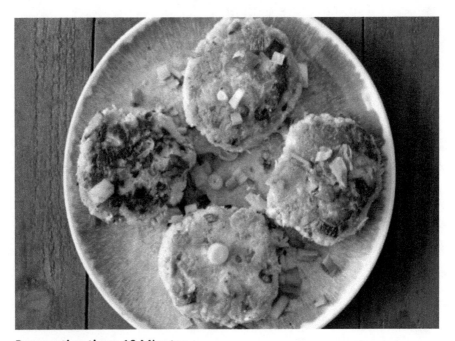

Preparation time: 10 Minutes

Cooking time: 10 Minutes

Servings: 8

Ingredients:

- 20oz. Canned tuna flakes
- ¼ Cup almond flour
- 1 Egg, beaten
- 2 Tablespoons fresh dill, chopped
- 2 Stalks green onion, chopped

- Salt and pepper to taste
- 1 Tablespoon lemon zest
- ¼ Cup mayonnaise
- 1 Tablespoon lemon juice
- 2 Tablespoons avocado oil

Directions:

1. Combine all the ingredients except avocado oil, lemon juice, and avocado oil in a large bowl.
2. Form 8 patties from the mixture.
3. In a pan over medium heat, add the oil.
4. Once the oil starts to sizzle, cook the tuna patties for 3 to 4 minutes per side.
5. Drain each patty on a paper towel.
6. Spread mayo on top and drizzle with lemon juice before serving.

Nutrition:

- Calories: 101
- Total Fat: 4.9g
- Saturated Fat: 1.2g
- Cholesterol: 47mg
- Sodium: 243mg
- Total Carbohydrate: 3.1g
- Dietary Fiber: 0.5g
- Total Sugars: 0.7g
- Protein: 12.3g
- Potassium: 60mg

Grilled Mahi Mahi with Lemon Butter Sauce

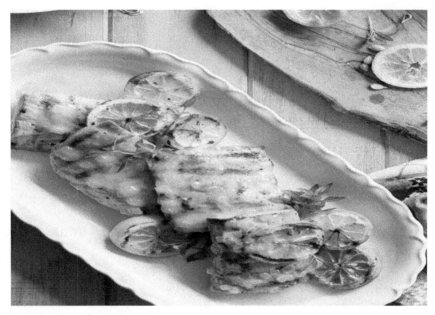

Preparation time: 20 Minutes

Cooking time: 10 Minutes

Servings: 6

Ingredients:

- 6 Mahi mahi fillets
- Salt and pepper to taste
- 2 Tablespoons olive oil
- 6 Tablespoons butter
- ¼ Onion, minced

- ½ Teaspoon garlic, minced
- ¼ Cup chicken stock
- 1 Tablespoon lemon juice

Directions:

1. Preheat your grill to medium heat.
2. Season fish fillets with salt and pepper.
3. Coat both sides with olive oil.
4. Grill for 3 to 4 minutes per side.
5. Place fish on a serving platter.
6. In a pan over medium heat, add the butter and let it melt.
7. Add the onion and sauté for 2 minutes.
8. Add the garlic and cook for 30 seconds.
9. Pour in the chicken stock.
10. Simmer until the stock has been reduced to half.
11. Add the lemon juice.
12. Pour the sauce over the grilled fish fillets.

Nutrition:

- Calories: 234 Total Fat: 17.2g
- Saturated Fat: 8.3g Cholesterol: 117mg
- Sodium: 242mg Total Carbohydrate: 0.6g
- Dietary Fiber: 0.1g Total Sugars: 0.3g
- Protein: 19.1g Potassium: 385mg

Shrimp Scampi

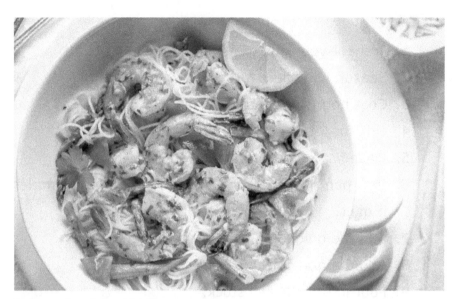

Preparation time: 15 Minutes

Cooking time: 10 Minutes

Servings: 6

Ingredients:

- 2 Tablespoons olive oil
- 2 Tablespoons butter
- 1 Tablespoon garlic, minced
- ½ Cup dry white wine
- ¼ Teaspoon red pepper flakes
- Salt and pepper to taste
- 2lb. Large shrimp, peeled and deveined
- ¼ Cup fresh parsley, chopped

- 1 Teaspoon lemon zest
- 2 Tablespoons lemon juice
- 3 Cups spaghetti squash, cooked

Directions:

1. In a pan over medium heat, add the oil and butter.
2. Cook the garlic for 2 minutes.
3. Pour in the wine.
4. Add the red pepper flakes, salt, and pepper.
5. Cook for 2 minutes.
6. Add the shrimp.
7. Cook for 2 to 3 minutes.
8. Remove from the stove.
9. Add the parsley, lemon zest, and lemon juice.
10. Serve on top of spaghetti squash.

Nutrition:

- Calories: 232 Total Fat: 8.9g
- Saturated Fat: 3.2g Cholesterol: 226mg
- Sodium: 229mg Total Carbohydrate: 7.6g
- Dietary Fiber: 0.2g Total Sugars: 0.3g
- Protein: 28.9g Potassium: 104mg

Dinner Recipes

Quick Pumpkin Soup

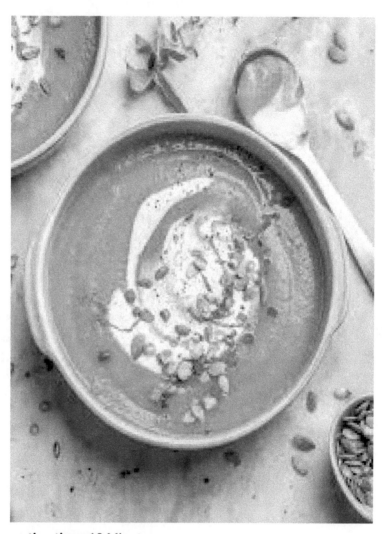

Preparation time: 10 Minutes

Cooking time: 20 Minutes

Servings: 4-6

Ingredients:

- 1 Cup of coconut milk
- 2 Cups chicken broth
- 6 Cups baked pumpkin
- 1 Tsp. garlic powder
- 1 Tsp. ground cinnamon
- 1 Tsp. dried ginger
- 1 Tsp. nutmeg
- 1 Tsp. paprika
- Salt and pepper, to taste
- Sour cream or coconut yogurt, for topping
- Pumpkin seeds, toasted, for topping

Directions:

1. Combine the coconut milk, broth, baked pumpkin, and spices in a soup pan (use medium heat). Stir occasionally and simmer for 15 minutes.
2. With an immersion blender, blend the soup mix for 1 minute.
3. Top with sour cream or coconut yogurt and pumpkin seeds.

Nutrition:

- Calories: 123 Fat: 9.8g
- Carbs: 8.1g Protein: 3.1g

Fresh Avocado Soup

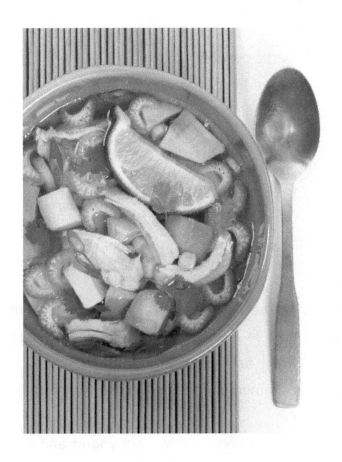

Preparation time: 5 Minutes

Cooking time: 10 Minutes

Servings: 2

Ingredients:

- 1 Ripe avocado
- 2 Romaine lettuce leaves, washed and chopped
- 1 Cup coconut milk, chilled
- 1 Tbsp. lime juice
- 20 Fresh mint leaves
- Salt, to taste

Directions:

1. Mix all your ingredients thoroughly in a blender.
2. Chill in the fridge for 5-10 minutes.

Nutrition:

- Calories: 280 Fat: 26g
- Carbs: 12g Protein: 4g

Creamy Garlic Chicken

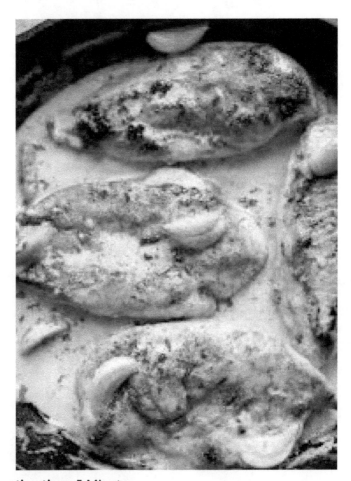

Preparation time: 5 Minutes

Cooking time: 15 Minutes

Servings: 4

Ingredients:

- 4 Chicken breasts, finely sliced
- 1 Tsp garlic powder

- 1 Tsp. paprika
- 2 Tbsp. butter
- 1 Tsp. salt
- 1 Cup heavy cream
- ½ Cup sun-dried tomatoes
- 2 Cloves garlic, minced
- 1 Cup spinach, chopped

Directions:

1. Blend the paprika, garlic powder, and salt and sprinkle over both sides of the chicken.
2. Melt the butter in a frying pan (choose medium heat). Add the chicken breast and fry for 5 minutes on each side. Set aside.
3. Add the heavy cream, sun-dried tomatoes, and garlic to the pan and whisk well to combine—Cook for 2 minutes. Add spinach and sauté for an additional 3 minutes. Return the chicken to the pan and cover with the sauce.

Nutrition: Calories: 280 Fat: 26g

- Carbohydrates: 12g Protein: 4g

Garlicky Pork Shoulder

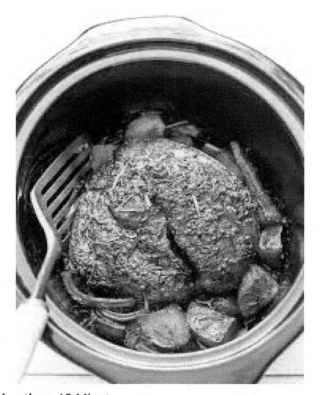

Preparation time: 15 Minutes

Cooking time: 6 Hours

Servings: 10

Ingredients:

- 1 Garlic head, peeled and crushed
- ¼ C. fresh rosemary, minced
- 2 Tbsp. fresh lemon juice
- 2 Tbsp. balsamic vinegar

- 1 (4-lb.) Pork shoulder

Directions:

1. In a bowl, add all the ingredients except pork shoulder and mix well.
2. In a large roasting pan, place the pork shoulder and generously coat with the marinade.
3. With a large plastic wrap, cover the roasting pan and refrigerate to marinate for at least 1-2 hours.
4. Remove the roasting pan from the refrigerator.
5. Remove the plastic wrap from the roasting pan and keep it at room temperature for 1 hour.
6. Preheat the oven to 2750 F.
7. Place the roasting pan into the oven and roast for about 6 hours.
8. Remove from the oven and place pork shoulder onto a cutting board for about 30 minutes.
9. With a sharp knife, cut the pork shoulder into desired size slices and serve.

Nutrition:

- Calories per serving: 502
- Carbohydrates: 2g Protein: 42.5g
- Fat: 39.1g Sugar: 0.1g
- Sodium: 125mg Fiber: 0.7g

Rosemary Pork Roast

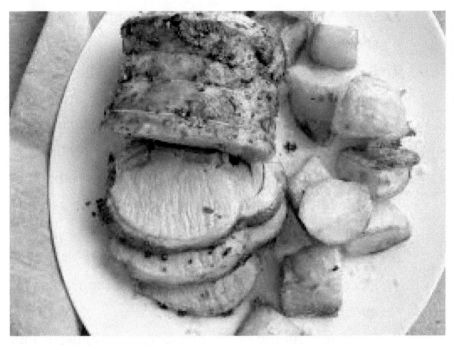

Preparation time: 15 Minutes

Cooking time: 1 Hour

Servings: 6

Ingredients:

- 1 Tbsp. dried rosemary, crushed
- 3 Garlic cloves, minced
- Salt and freshly ground black pepper, to taste
- 2lb. Boneless pork loin roast
- ¼ C. olive oil
- 1/3 C. homemade chicken broth

Directions:

1. Preheat the oven to 3500 F. Lightly grease a roasting pan. In a small bowl, add rosemary, garlic, salt, black pepper, and with the back of a spoon, crush the mixture to form a paste.
2. With a sharp knife, pierce the pork loin at many places.
3. Press half of the rosemary mixture into the cuts.
4. Add oil in the bowl with the remaining rosemary mixture and stir to combine.
5. Rub the pork with rosemary mixture generously. Arrange the pork loin into the prepared roasting pan. Roast for about 1 hour, flipping and coating with the pan juices occasionally.
6. Remove the roasting pan from the oven. Transfer the pork to a serving platter.
7. Place the roasting pan over medium heat.
8. Add the broth and cook for about 3-5 minutes, stirring to lose the brown bits from the pan. Pour sauce over pork and serve.

Nutrition:

- Calories per serving: 294
- Carbohydrates: 0.9g Protein: 40g
- Fat: 13.9g Sugar: 0.1g
- Sodium: 156mg Fiber: 0.3g

Persian Chicken

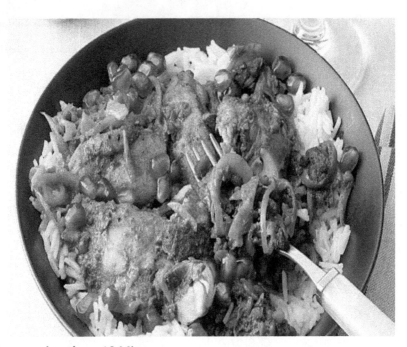

Preparation time: 10 Minutes

Cooking time: 20 Minutes

Servings: 6

Ingredients: 1/2 Small sweet onion,

- 1/4 Cup freshly squeezed lemon juice
- 1 Tablespoon dried oregano
- 1/2 Tablespoon of sweet paprika,
- 1/2 Tablespoon of ground cumin
- 1/2 Cup olive oil
- 6 Boneless, skinless chicken thighs

Directions:

1. Put the vegetables in a blender. Mix it well.
2. Put the olive while the motor is running.
3. In a sealable bag for the freezer, place the chicken thighs and put the mixture in the sealable bag. Refrigerate it for 2 hours, while turning it two times. Remove the marinade thighs and discard the additional marinade. Preheat the barbecue to medium. Grill the chicken, turning once or until the inner part is well done.

Nutrition: Fat: 21g Carbohydrates: 3g

- Potassium: 220mg Sodium: 86mg
- Protein: 22g

Pesto Pork Chops

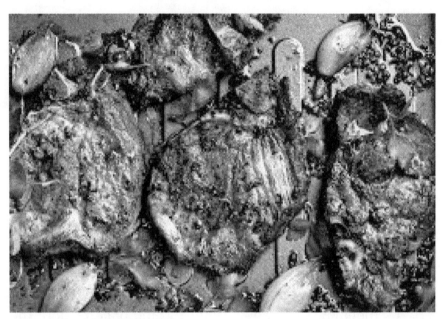

Preparation time: 20 Minutes

Cooking time: 20 Minutes

Servings: 3

Ingredients:

- 3 (3-ounce) Top-flood pork chops, boneless, fat
- 8 Tablespoons Herb Pesto (here)
- 1/2 Cup bread crumbs
- 1 Tablespoon olive oil

Directions:

1. Preheat the oven to 360 ° F. Cover a foil baker's sheet; set aside.

2. Rub one tablespoon of pesto evenly across each pork chop on both sides.

3. Every pork chop in the crumbs of bread is lightly dredged.

4. Heat the oil in a medium-high heat large skillet. Brown the pork chops for about 6 minutes on each side.

5. Place on the baking sheet the pork chops. Bake until the pork reaches 136 ° F in the center for about 10 minutes.

Nutrition: Fat: 8g Carbohydrates: 10g

- Phosphorus: 188mg Potassium: 220mg
- Sodium: 138mg Protein: 23g

Roasted Red Pepper and Eggplant Soup

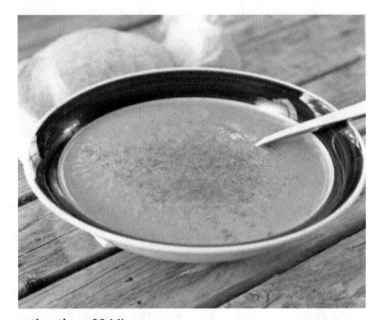

Preparation time: 20 Minutes

Cooking time: 40 Minutes

Servings: 6

Ingredients:

- 1 Small sweet onion, cut into quarters
- 2 Small red peppers, halved
- 2 Cups of eggplant
- 2 Garlic cloves, crushed
- 1 Cup of olive oil
- 1 Cup of Easy Chicken Stock
- Water
- 1/4 Cup of chopped fresh basil

Directions:

1. Preheat the oven to 360 ° F. In a large ovenproof baking dish, place the onions, red peppers, eggplant, and garlic.
2. Add the olive oil to the vegetables.
3. Roast the vegetables. For about 40 minutes or until slightly charred and soft.
4. Slightly cool the vegetables and remove the peppers from the skin.
5. In a food processor (or in a large bowl, using a handheld immersion blender), purée the vegetables with the chicken stock. Move the soup to a large pot and add sufficient water to achieve the desired thickness. Heat the soup and add the basil to a simmer. Season and serve with pepper.

Nutrition: Fat: 2g Carbohydrates: 8g

- Phosphorus: 33mg Potassium: 188mg
- Sodium: 86mg Protein: 2g

Cilantro-Lime Flounder

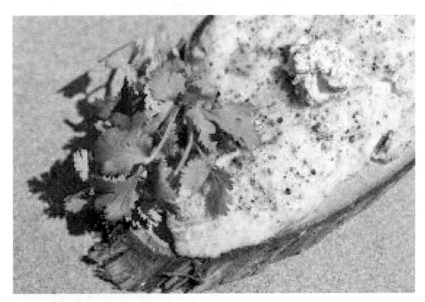

Preparation time: 20 Minutes

Cooking time: 6 Minutes

Servings: 3

Ingredients:

- 1/4 Cup homemade mayonnaise
- 1 Lime juice Zest
- 1 1/2 Cup fresh cilantro
- 3 (3-ounce) Flounder fillets

Directions:

1. Preheat the oven to 300 ° F. Stir the mayonnaise, lime juice, lime zest, and cilantro in a small bowl.

2. Place three pieces of foil on a clean work surface, about 8x8 inches square. In the center of each square, place a flounder fillet.

3. Top the fillets with the mixture of mayonnaise evenly. Season the flounder with the pepper. Fold the foil sides over the fish, create a snug packet, and place on a baking sheet the foil packets. Bake the fish for three to six minutes. Unfold and display the boxes.

Nutrition: Fat: 3g Carbohydrates: 2g

- Phosphorus: 208mg Potassium: 138mg
- Sodium: 268mg Protein: 12g

Dana Roberts

Dessert Recipes

Snickerdoodle Muffins

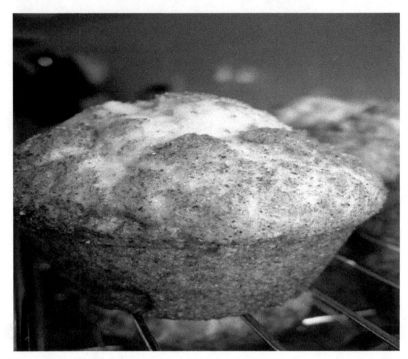

Preparation time: 10 Minutes

Cooking time: 12 Minutes

Servings: 6

Ingredients:

- 6 2/3 Tbsp. coconut flour
- 1/2 Egg
- 1 Tbsp. butter, unsalted, melted
- 1 1/3 Tbsp. whipping cream
- 1 Tbsp. almond milk, unsweetened

Others:

- 1 1/3 Tbsp. erythritol sweetener and more for topping
- 1/4 Tsp. baking powder
- 1/4 Tsp. ground cinnamon and more for topping
- 1/4 Tsp. vanilla extract, unsweetened

Directions:

1. Turn on the oven, set it to 350 degrees F and let it preheat.
2. Meanwhile, take a medium bowl, place flour in it, add cinnamon and baking powder. Stir until combined.
3. Take a separate bowl, place the half egg in it, add butter, sour cream, milk, vanilla, and whisk until blended.
4. Whisk the flour mixture until a smooth batter is obtained, divide the batter evenly between two silicon muffin cups, and then sprinkle cinnamon and sweetener on top.
5. Bake the muffins for 10 to 12 minutes until firm, and then the top has turned golden brown and then serve and enjoy!

Nutrition:

- Calories: 299 Fat: 13.2g
- Fiber: 10.5g Carbohydrates:4.1g
- Protein: 3.8g

Egg Custard

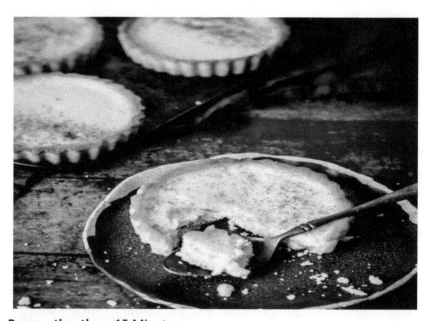

Preparation time: 15 Minutes

Cooking time: 55 Minutes

Servings: 8

Ingredients:

- 5 Organic eggs
- Salt, as required
- ½ Cup Yacon syrup
- 20 Ounces unsweetened almond milk
- ¼ Teaspoon ground ginger
- ¼ Teaspoon ground cinnamon
- ¼ Teaspoon ground nutmeg
- ¼ Teaspoon ground cardamom
- 1/8 Teaspoon ground cloves
- 1/8 Teaspoon ground allspice

Directions:

1. Preheat your oven to 325ºF.
2. Grease 8 small ramekins.
3. In a bowl, add the eggs and salt and beat well.
4. Arrange a sieve over a medium bowl.
5. Through a sieve, strain the egg mixture into a bowl.
6. Add the Yacon syrup to the eggs and stir to combine.
7. Add the almond milk and spices and beat until well combined.
8. Transfer the mixture into prepared ramekins.
9. Now, place ramekins in a large baking dish.
10. Add hot water in the baking dish about 2-inch high around the ramekins.
11. Place the baking dish in the oven and bake for about 30–40 minutes or until a toothpick inserted in the center comes out clean.
12. Remove ramekins from the oven and set aside to cool.
13. Refrigerate to chill before serving.

Nutrition:

- Calories: 77
- Fat: 3.8g
- Carbs: 6g
- Cholesterol: 102mg
- Sodium: 116mg
- Fiber: 0.5g
- Sugar: 3.7g
- Protein: 3.8g

Mocha Ice Cream

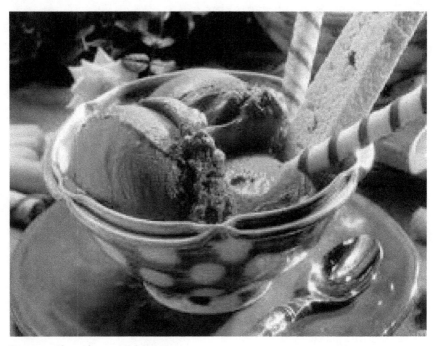

Preparation time: 15 Minutes

Cooking time: 15 Minutes

Servings: 2

Ingredients:

- 1 Cup unsweetened coconut milk
- ¼ Cup heavy cream
- 2 Tablespoons granulated erythritol
- 15 Drops liquid stevia
- 2 Tablespoons cacao powder
- 1 Tablespoon instant coffee

- ¼ Teaspoon xanthan gum

Directions:

1. In a container, add the ingredients (except xanthan gum), and with an immersion blender, blend until well combined.
2. Slowly add the xanthan gum and blend until a slightly thicker mixture is formed.
3. Transfer the mixture into the ice cream maker and process according to the manufacturer's instructions.
4. Now, transfer the ice cream into an airtight container and freeze for at least 4–5 hours before serving.

Nutrition:

- Calories: 246 Carbs: 6.2g
- Fat: 23.1g Cholesterol: 21mg
- Sodium: 52mg Fiber: 2g
- Sugar: 3g
- Protein: 2.8g

Condiment Recipes

Thai Peanut Sauce

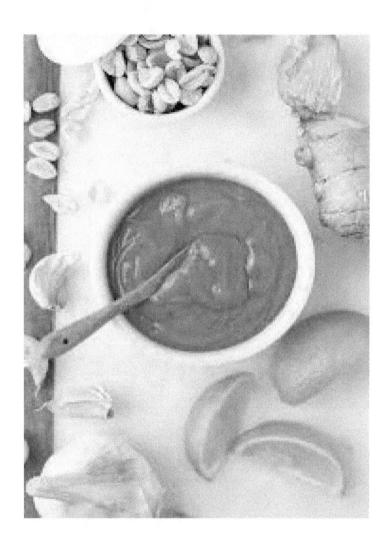

Preparation time: 5 Minutes

Cooking time: 0 Minutes

Servings: 3

Ingredients:

- 2 Tbsp. Apple Cider Vinegar
- ¼ Cup Thai Red Curry Paste
- 1 Cup Peanut Butter
- 1 ½ Cup Coconut Milk
- 1 Tbsp. Lime Juice
- ¼ Cup Brown Sugar
- 2 Tbsp. Soy Sauce

Directions:

1. For a quick and easy sauce, simply place everything into a food processor and meld until soft. Be sure you keep any sauce and dressing in the fridge to keep fresh!

Nutrition:

- Calories: 100 Carbs: 9g
- Fat: 7g Protein: 1g

General Tso Sauce

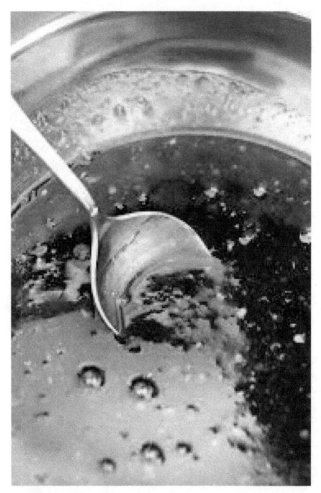

Preparation time: 5 Minutes

Cooking time: 10 Minutes

Servings: 4

Ingredients:

- ¼ Cup rice vinegar
- ½ Cup water
- 1 ½ tablespoon sriracha sauce
- ¼ Cup soy sauce
- 1 ½ Tablespoon corn starch
- ½ Cup sugar

Directions:

1. General Tso Sauce is a classic, and you can now make a healthier version of it! All you have to do is take out your saucepan and place all of the ingredients in.

2. Once in place, bring everything over medium heat and whisk together for ten minutes or until the sauce begins to get thick.

3. Finally, remove from the heat and enjoy!

Nutrition:

- Calories: 80 Carbs: 11g
- Fat: 3g Protein: 2g

Dana Roberts

Smoothies Recipes

Tropical Green Paleo Smoothie

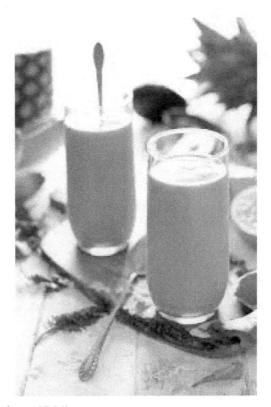

Preparation time: 15 Minutes

Cooking time: 0 Minutes

Servings: 5

Ingredients:

- Spinach. 3 cups (Kale, or a blend of small leafy greens, packed)
- Whole Banana. 1 (Peeled)
- Whole Orange. 1 (Peeled)
- Pineapple. 1-½ cup (Cubed)
- Coconut Milk. 1 cup

- Whole Avocado. ½ (pitted and skin removed)
- Crushed Ice. 2 cups
- Wild Orange Essential Oil. 3 drops (optional)
- Dried Coconut Chip. 10 pieces (optional)
- Dried Coconut Chips for Topping (optional)
- Pure Maple Syrup. 1 Tablespoon (optional, depends on the sweetness of fruit)
- Chia Seeds for Topping. One teaspoon (optional)

Directions:

1. Add all the ingredients minus the chia seeds and coconut chips in a high-speed blender. Blend for about 2 minutes, until creamy and smooth.
2. Transfer mixture to serving glasses and top with the chia seeds and coconut seeds. It can be refrigerated for up to 3 days. Stir quickly to recombine if placed in the fridge.

Nutrition:

- Calories per serving: 33
- Carbohydrates: 8.5g
- Protein: 2.2g
- Fat: 0.4g
- Sugar: 4.3g
- Sodium: 225mg
- Fiber: 1.9g

Vegan Banana Avocado Green Smoothie Bowl with Blueberries

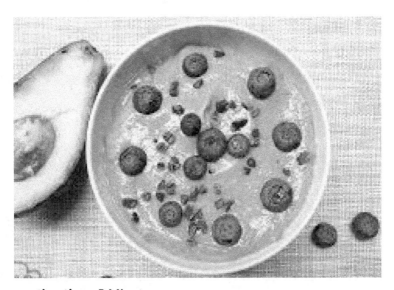

Preparation time: 5 Minutes

Cooking time: 0 Minutes

Servings: 1

Ingredients:

For the Smoothie:

- Fresh Baby Spinach. 60 grams
- Whole Avocado. ½
- Whole Peach. 1
- Whole Banana. ½
- Rolled Oats. 2 Tablespoons
- Peanut Butter. 1 Tablespoon
- Coconut Water. 3 Tablespoons

For the Topping:

1. Whole Blueberries. 12
2. Cacao Nibs. 1 teaspoon

Directions:

1. Add all the smoothie ingredients to your blender. Blend until creamy and smooth, about 30 seconds.
2. Pour into a bowl and add toppings.
3. Enjoy!

Nutrition:

- Calories per serving: 414
- Carbohydrates: 10.8g
- Protein: 12.5g
- Fat: 35.7g
- Sugar: 0.6g
- Sodium: 188mg
- Fiber: 4.8g

Kale Strawberry Green Smoothie Bowl

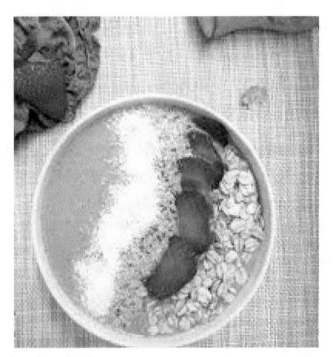

Preparation time: 8 Minutes

Cooking time: 0 Minutes

Servings: 1

Ingredients:

For the Smoothie:

- Whole Strawberries. 2
- Zucchini. 2 ounces
- Kale. 1 cup
- Sliced Cucumber. 1.4 ounces

- Whole Banana. ½
- Dairy-Free Milk. 4 tablespoons

For the Topping:

- Whole Strawberry. 1
- Hemp Hearts. ½ Tablespoon
- Shredded Coconut. 1 Tablespoon
- Whole Oats. 2 Tablespoons

Directions:

1. Add all the smoothie ingredients to a high-speed blender. Blend for about 2 minutes, until it is creamy and smooth.
2. Transfer the mixture to serving bowls and add the toppings.

Nutrition:

- Calories per serving: 326
- Carbohydrates: 8.2g
- Protein: 7.8g Fat: 29.4g
- Sugar: 0.3g Sodium: 126mg
- Fiber: 4.1g

Dana Roberts

Salad Recipes

Potluck Lamb Salad

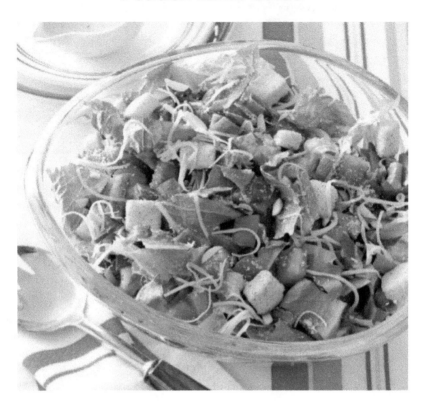

Preparation time: 20 Minutes

Cooking time: 10 Minutes

Servings: 4

Ingredients:

- 2 Tbsp. olive oil, divided
- 12oz. Grass-fed lamb leg steaks, trimmed
- Salt and freshly ground black pepper, to taste
- 6½oz. halloumi cheese, cut into thick slices
- 2 Jarred roasted red bell peppers, sliced thinly

- 2 Cucumbers, cut into thin ribbons
- 3 C. fresh baby spinach
- 2 Tbsp. balsamic vinegar

Directions:

1. In a skillet, heat one tablespoon of the oil over medium-high heat and cook the lamb steaks for about 4-5 minutes per side or until desired doneness. Transfer the lamb steaks onto a cutting board for about 5 minutes. Then cut the lamb steaks into thin slices.

2. In the same skillet, add halloumi and cook for about 1-2 minutes per side or until golden. In a salad bowl, add the lamb, haloumi, bell pepper, cucumber, salad leaves, vinegar, and remaining oil and toss to combine. Serve immediately.

Nutrition:

- Calories: 420 Carbohydrates: 8g
- Protein: 35.4g Fat: 27.2g
- Sugar: 4g Sodium: 417mg Fiber: 1.3g

Spring Supper Salad

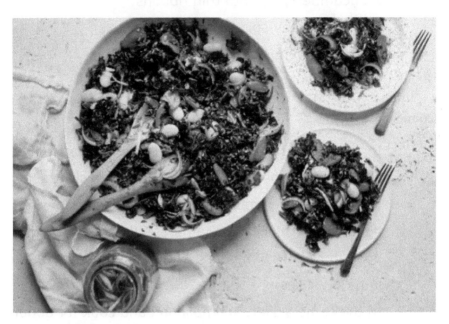

Preparation time: 15 Minutes

Cooking time: 5 Minutes

Servings: 5

Ingredients:

For the salad:

- 1 lb. Fresh asparagus, trimmed and cut into 1-inch pieces
- ½ lb. Smoked salmon, cut into bite-sized pieces
- 2 Heads red leaf lettuce, torn
- ¼ C. pecans, toasted and chopped

For dressing:

- ¼ C. olive oil - 2 Tbsp. fresh lemon juice
- 1 Tsp. Dijon mustard
- Salt and freshly ground black pepper, to taste

Directions:

1. In a pan of boiling water, add the asparagus and cook for about 5 minutes.
2. Drain the asparagus well. In a serving bowl, add the asparagus and remaining salad ingredients and mix.
3. In another bowl, add all the dressing ingredients and beat until well combined.
4. Place the dressing over salad and gently toss to coat well. Serve immediately.

Nutrition:

- Calories: 223 Carbohydrates: 8.5g
- Protein: 11.7g Fat: 17.2g
- Sugar: 3.4g Sodium: 960mg Fiber: 3.5g

Chicken-of-Sea Salad

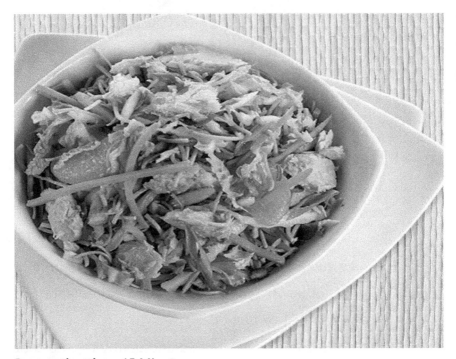

Preparation time: 15 Minutes

Cooking time: 5 Minutes

Servings: 6

Ingredients:

- 2 (6-oz.) cans olive oil-packed tuna, drained
- 2 (6-oz.) cans water-packed tuna, drained
- ¾ C. mayonnaise
- 2 Celery stalks, chopped
- ¼ of onion, chopped
- 1 Tbsp. fresh lime juice

- 2 Tbsp. mustard
- Freshly ground black pepper, to taste
- 6 C. fresh baby arugula

Directions:

1. In a large bowl, add all the ingredients except arugula and gently stir to combine.
2. Divide arugula onto serving plates and top with tuna mixture.
3. Serve immediately.

Nutrition:

- Calories: 325 Carbohydrates: 2.7g
- Protein: 27.4g Fat: 22.2g
- Sugar: 0.9g Sodium: 389mg Fiber: 1.1g

Sweet Potato Salad

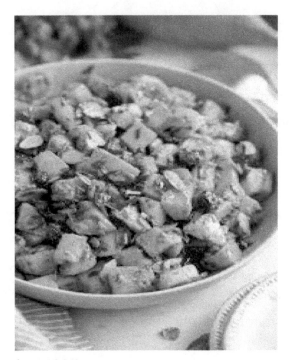

Preparation time: 10 Minutes

Cooking time: 10 Minutes

Servings: 3

Ingredients:

- 2 Teaspoons olive oil
- 1 Sweet potato, spiralized
- 1 Apple, cored and spiralized
- 3 Tablespoons almonds, toasted and sliced
- Salt, to taste
- 3 Cups spinach, torn

For the salad dressing:

- 1 Teaspoon apple cider vinegar
- 2 Tablespoons apple juice
- 1 Tablespoon almond butter, melted
- ½ Teaspoon ginger, minced
- 1½ Teaspoons mustard
- 1 Tablespoon olive oil

Directions:

1. In a bowl, mix the vinegar with the apple juice, almond butter, ginger, mustard, and one tablespoon oil and whisk.
2. Heat a pan with the two teaspoons oil over medium-high heat, add the sweet potato noodles, stir, cook for 7 minutes and transfer to a bowl.
3. Add the rest of the ingredients and the dressing, toss and serve.

Nutrition:

- Calories per serving: 500
- Carbohydrates: 7g
- Protein: 8g
- Fat: 2g
- Sugar: 0.3g
- Sodium: 434mg
- Fiber: 0g

Dana Roberts

Appetizers and Snacks

Spiced Jalapeno Bites with Tomato

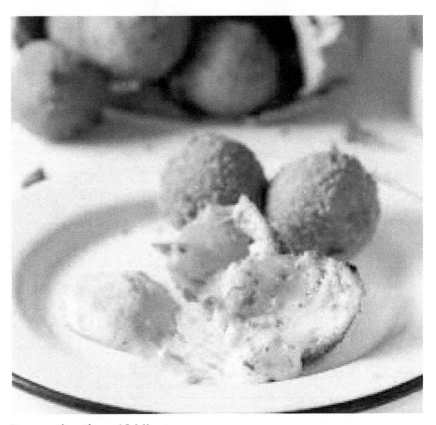

Preparation time: 10 Minutes

Cooking time: 0 Minutes

Servings: 4

Ingredients:

- 1 Cup turkey ham, chopped
- 1/4 Jalapeño pepper, minced
- 1/4 Cup mayonnaise
- 1/3 Tablespoon Dijon mustard
- 4 Tomatoes, sliced

- Salt and black pepper, to taste
- 1 Tablespoon parsley, chopped

Directions:

1. In a bowl, mix the turkey ham, jalapeño pepper, mayo, mustard, salt, and pepper.
2. Spread out the tomato slices on four serving plates, then top each plate with a spoonful turkey ham mixture.
3. Serve garnished with chopped parsley.

Nutrition: Calories: 250 Fat: 14.1g

- Fiber: 3.7g Carbohydrates: 4.1g
- Protein: 18.9g

Coconut Crab Cakes

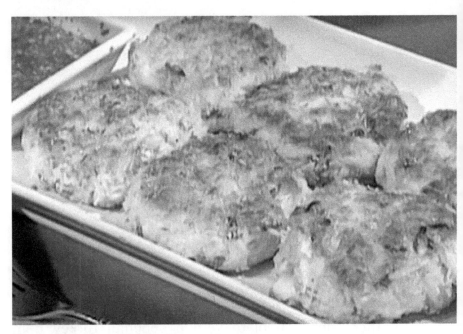

Preparation time: 20 Minutes

Cooking time: 25 Minutes

Servings: 4

Ingredients:

- 1 Tablespoon of minced garlic
- 2 Pasteurized eggs
- 2 Teaspoons of coconut oil
- 3/4 Cup of coconut flakes
- 3/4 Cup chopped spinach
- 1/4 Pound crabmeat
- 1/4 Cup of chopped leek
- 1/2 Cup extra virgin olive oil
- 1/2 Teaspoon of pepper

- 1/4 Onion diced
- Salt

Directions:

1. Pour the crabmeat into a bowl, then add in the coconut flakes and mix well.
2. Whisk eggs in a bowl, then mix in leek and spinach.
3. Season the egg mixture with pepper, two pinches of salt, and garlic.
4. Then, pour the eggs into the crab and stir well.
5. Preheat a pan, heat extra virgin olive, and fry the crab evenly from each side until golden brown. Remove from the pan and serve hot.

Nutrition:

- Calories: 254 Fat: 9.5g
- Fiber: 5.4g Carbohydrates: 4.1g
- Protein: 8.9g

Tuna Cakes

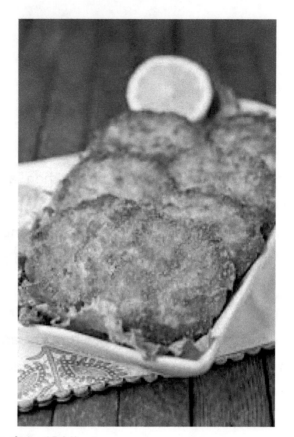

Preparation time: 15 Minutes

Cooking time: 10 Minutes

Servings: 2

Ingredients:

- 1 (15-ounce) can water-packed tuna, drained
- 1/2 Celery stalk, chopped
- 2 Tablespoon fresh parsley, chopped
- 1 Teaspoon fresh dill, chopped
- 2 Tablespoons walnuts, chopped

- 2 Tablespoons mayonnaise
- 1 Organic egg, beaten
- 1 Tablespoon butter
- 3 Cups lettuce

Directions:

1. For burgers: Add all ingredients (except the butter and lettuce) in a bowl and mix until well combined.
2. Make two equal-sized patties from the mixture.
3. Melt some butter and cook the patties for about 2–3 minutes.
4. Carefully flip the side and cook for about 2–3 minutes.
5. Divide the lettuce onto serving plates.
6. Top each plate with one burger and serve.

Nutrition:

- Calories: 267 Fat: 12.5g
- Fiber: 9.4g Carbohydrates:3.8g
- Protein: 11.5g

Tempura Zucchini with Cream Cheese Dip

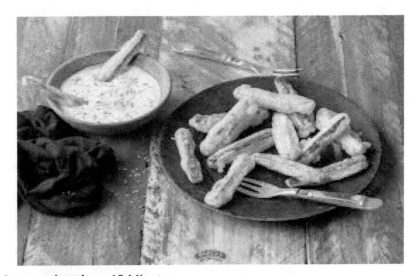

Preparation time: 15 Minutes

Cooking time: 15 Minutes

Servings: 4

Ingredients:

For Tempura zucchinis:

- 1 1/2 Cups (200 g) almond flour
- 2 Tbsp. heavy cream
- 1 Tsp. salt
- 2 Tbsp. olive oil + extra for frying
- 1 1/4 Cups (300 ml) water
- 1/2 Tbsp. sugar-free maple syrup
- 2 Large zucchinis, cut into 1-inch thick strips

For Cream cheese dip:

- 8oz. Cream cheese, room temperature
- 1/2 Cup (113 g) sour cream

- 1 Tsp. Taco seasoning
- 1 Scallion, chopped
- 1 Green chili, deseeded and minced

Directions:

Tempura zucchinis:

1. In a bowl, mix the almond flour, heavy cream, salt, peanut oil, water, and maple syrup.
2. Dredge the zucchini strips in the mixture until well-coated.
3. Heat about four tablespoons of olive oil in a non-stick skillet.
4. Working in batches, use tongs to remove the zucchinis (draining extra liquid) into the oil.
5. Fry per side for 1 to 2 minutes and remove the zucchinis onto a paper towel-lined plate to drain grease.
6. Enjoy the zucchinis.

Cream cheese dip:

1. In a bowl or container, the cream cheese, taco seasoning, sour cream, scallion, and green chili must be mixed,
2. Serve the tempura zucchinis with the cream cheese dip.

Nutrition:

- Calories: 316 Fat: 8.4g
- Fiber: 9.3g Carbohydrates: 4.1g
- Protein: 5.1g

Bacon and Feta Skewers

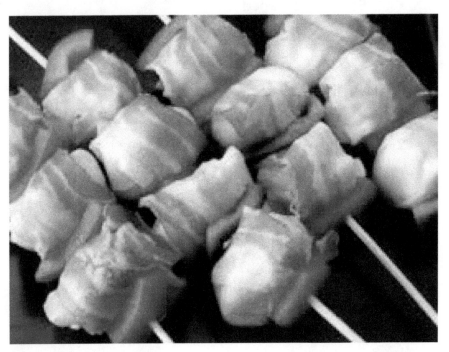

Preparation time: 15 Minutes

Cooking time: 10 Minutes

Servings: 4

Ingredients:

- 2 lb. Feta cheese, cut into 8 cubes
- 8 Bacon slices
- 4 Bamboo skewers, soaked
- 1 Zucchini, cut into 8 bite-size cubes
- Salt and black pepper to taste
- 3 Tbsp. almond oil for brushing

Directions:

1. Wrap each feta cube with a bacon slice.
2. Thread one wrapped feta on a skewer; add a zucchini cube, then another wrapped feta, and another zucchini.
3. Repeat the threading process with the remaining skewers.
4. Preheat a grill pan to medium heat, generously brush with the avocado oil and grill the skewer on both sides for 3 to 4 minutes per side or until the set is golden brown and the bacon cooked.
5. Serve afterward with the tomato salsa.

Nutrition:

- Calories: 290 Fat: 15.1g
- Fiber: 4.2g
- Carbohydrates: 4.1g
- Protein: 11.8g

Avocado and Prosciutto Deviled Eggs

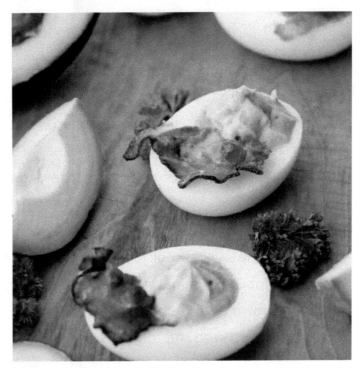

Preparation time: 20 Minutes

Cooking time: 10 Minutes

Servings: 4

Ingredients:

- 4 Eggs
- Ice bath
- 4 Prosciutto slices, chopped
- 1 Avocado, pitted and peeled
- 1 Tbsp. mustard
- 1 Tsp. plain vinegar
- 1 Tbsp. heavy cream
- 1 Tbsp. chopped fresh cilantro
- Salt and black pepper to taste
- 1/2 Cup (113 g) mayonnaise

- 1 Tbsp. coconut cream
- 1/4 Tsp. cayenne pepper
- 1 Tbsp. avocado oil
- 1 Tbsp. chopped fresh parsley

Directions:

1. Boil the eggs for 8 minutes.
2. Remove the eggs into the ice bath, sit for 3 minutes, and then peel the eggs.
3. Slice the eggs lengthwise into halves and empty the egg yolks into a bowl.
4. Arrange the egg whites on a plate with the hole side facing upwards.
5. While the eggs are cooked, heat a non-stick skillet over medium heat and cook the prosciutto for 5 to 8 minutes.
6. Remove the prosciutto onto a paper towel-lined plate to drain grease.
7. Put the avocado slices into the egg yolks and mash both ingredients with a fork until smooth.
8. Mix in the mustard, vinegar, heavy cream, cilantro, salt, and black pepper until well-blended.
9. Spoon the mixture into a piping bag and press the mixture into the egg holes until well-filled.
10. In a bowl, whisk the mayonnaise, coconut cream, cayenne pepper, and avocado oil.
11. On serving plates, spoon some of the mayonnaise sauce and slightly smear it in a circular movement. Top with the deviled eggs, scatter the prosciutto on top, and garnish with the parsley.
12. Enjoy immediately.

Nutrition:

- Calories: 265 Fat: 11.7g
- Fiber: 4.1g Carbohydrates: 3.1g
- Protein:7.9g

Chicken Club Lettuce Wraps

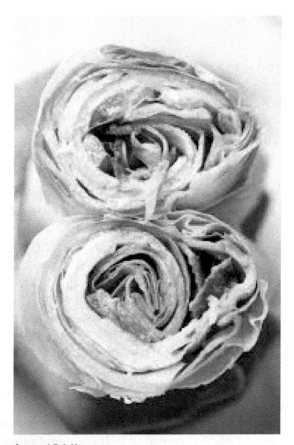

Preparation time: 15 Minutes

Cooking time: 15 Minutes

Servings: 1

Ingredients:

- 1 Head of iceberg lettuce with the core and outer leaves removed
- 1 Tbsp. of mayonnaise

- 6 Slices of organic chicken or turkey breast
- Bacon (2 cooked strips, halved)
- Tomato (just 2 slices)

Directions:

1. Line your working surface with a large slice of parchment paper.
2. Layer 6-8 large leaves of lettuce in the center of the paper to make a base of around 9-10 inches.
3. Spread the mayo in the center and lay with chicken or turkey, bacon, and tomato.
4. Starting with the end closest to you, roll the wrap like a jelly roll with the parchment paper as your guide. Keep it tight and halfway through, roll tuck in the ends of the wrap.
5. When it is completely wrapped, roll the rest of the parchment paper around it, and use a knife to cut it in half.

Nutrition:

- Calories: 179
- Fat: 4.1g
- Fiber: 9.7g
- Carbohydrates: 1.3g
- Protein: 8.5g

About the author

Dana Roberts is an author, nutritionist and mom of three beautiful princesses.

At the age of 38 she discovered that she had breast disease and this brought her a big hormonal imbalance.

At the age of 43 she noticed a gradual weight gain that prompted her to try different diets.

So many of these had little or no effect on her. After a few years, her body underwent drastic changes.

She gained a lot of weight, her breasts collapsed and a lot of stretch marks appeared. Not wanting to risk serious health problems, she discovered the ketogenic diet and decided to try it.

She began to notice that some foods gave her more energy and others weighed her down. Food addiction also influenced her diet because when she didn't bring awareness to her emotions, she reacted by eating.

She spent years fighting this addiction and finally found a way to overcome it and rediscover her former beauty, creating recipes that could fill both her stomach and her soul.

The book "Keto Diet Cookbook for women after 50" offers to all women the possibility to lose weight with a program based not only on diet, but also on the addiction that sometimes food creates.

CPSIA information can be obtained
at www.ICGtesting.com
Printed in the USA
BVHW090322230221
600781BV00006B/969